Christina Macdonald is an award-winning editor with a career in magazine journalism spanning more than 20 years. She is the former Editor-in-Chief of *Women's Running* magazine and is currently Online Editor of The Alzheimer's Show, for which she provides regular content on many different aspects of living with dementia. She is also author of the book *Run Yourself Fit*, and credits regular exercise with helping her remain positive while caring for her mother Hazel, who has vascular dementia. You can read her blogs and dementia articles at <www.alzheimersshow.co.uk>.

Overcoming Common Problems Series

Selected titles

A full list of titles is available from Sheldon Press,
36 Causton Street, London SW1P 4ST and on our website at
www.sheldonpress.co.uk

DEMENTIA CARE

A GUIDE

CHRISTINA MACDONALD

sheldon PRESS

First published in Great Britain in 2016

Sheldon Press
36 Causton Street
London SW1P 4ST
www.sheldonpress.co.uk

British Library Cataloguing-in-Publication Data
A catalogue record for this book is available from the British Library

ISBN 978–1–84709–399–8
eBook ISBN 978–1–84709–400–1

Typeset by Fakenham Prepress Solutions, Fakenham, Norfolk NR21 8NN
First printed in Great Britain by Ashford Colour Press
Subsequently digitally reprinted in Great Britain

eBook by Fakenham Prepress Solutions, Fakenham, Norfolk NR21 8NN
Produced on paper from sustainable forests

For Eddie, April and Alex.
Your support means everything

Contents

Acknowledgements

Age UK, The Alzheimer's Show, Alzheimer's Society, SweetTree Home Care Services, United Kingdom Homecare Association (UKHCA).

Special thanks: Colin Angel, Carole Broughton, Janice Coles, Sara Couchman, Vicki Hodgkinson, Rikki Lorenti, Stephen Lowe, Rob Stewart, Barry Sweetbaum, Nigel Ward, Vivien Ziwocha.

Note to the reader

This book is not intended to be a substitute for medical advice. All information is correct at the time of going to press.

Introduction

My mother was diagnosed with vascular dementia in 2009. Looking back, the warning signs were there a year or so before Mum's diagnosis. She started forgetting things and repeating questions. She got confused while carrying out routine tasks and began putting things in strange places. One day she got lost driving to the vet's, which was a very familiar journey for her. One morning, my father found the kettle in the fridge. She had increasingly frequent moments of confusion.

At the time, Mum was caring for my father, who was seriously ill, so it was easy to blame her confusion on the stress of being a full-time carer. When my father died, her problems became more apparent. This is not uncommon in a person with dementia after a bereavement. It could be because the person who died might have helped the person with dementia, so that the full impact of the illness was less apparent to others, or it could be that caring for a loved one gave the person with dementia a focus.

My mother knew that her memory was letting her down, but was reluctant to seek help. Eventually I persuaded her to visit the GP, who conducted a short memory test and then referred her for a blood test and a brain scan. The diagnosis was confirmed by the results of the scan but I don't think Mum quite understood what it meant and she had forgotten about it a few days later.

And so began a challenging journey of caring for Mum that still continues to this day.

I wish I'd known then what I know now – I'm sure if I'd understood more about dementia at the time I would have been more patient and understanding during some of the more difficult moments. Like a lot of people, I wrongly assumed that it only affected the memory, but it can also have a significant effect on moods and behaviour.

I'm not a medical expert and there are many good books that explore the physical effects of dementia. This book is written from hands-on, personal experience. It's the book I wish I'd been able to read back in 2009, when I knew very little. It wouldn't have solved every problem, but knowledge is power, and it would certainly have helped.

Each situation and person is unique, and it's impossible to predict every scenario you may experience. But I hope that some of my personal insights will help you to cope and also feel that someone else understands what you are experiencing. Even though you may feel isolated at times, I'd like to stress that you're not alone. There are organizations you can contact for help. Their details are at the back of this book.

Good luck with the journey ahead – you will learn much and hopefully this book will go some way to helping you cope and provide the best possible care for your parent or loved one. And if you'd like to get in touch and share your experiences, you can message me on Twitter @writefitchris.

Christina Macdonald

1

What is dementia?

If your parent or other loved one has just been diagnosed with dementia, you may have some knowledge of the symptoms. Most likely you've noticed him or her having memory problems. However, dementia is about more than just memory loss. The more you understand about it, the better placed you will be to cope with the challenges ahead.

The word 'dementia' is not a diagnosis. Rather, it's an umbrella term describing a set of symptoms such as memory loss, difficulties with language, thinking and solving problems. These symptoms occur when certain diseases or conditions affect the brain. Dementia is not a natural part of ageing, although the risk of developing it increases with age. At the time of writing, Alzheimer's Society estimates that there are 850,000 people in the UK living with dementia, most of them over 65, but there are more than 40,000 people with young onset dementia under this age.

Unfortunately, dementia is progressive and there is no cure. This means that a person's ability to remember things, communicate and understand will gradually decline. Over time, people will gradually lose their independence.

Dementia is on the increase. According to an Alzheimer's Society 2014 report, there will be one million people with dementia in the UK by 2025. The cost is significant. Alzheimer's Society says there are 670,000 carers in the UK for people with dementia and it is estimated to cost the UK economy £26 billion per year. Yet getting a diagnosis can be difficult. According to the Health and Social Care Information Centre, only 67.2 per cent of people in England receive a diagnosis. In Scotland, only 64 per cent are diagnosed according to Alzheimer's Scotland, 43.4 per cent in Wales according to Alzheimer's Society and 64.8 per cent in Northern Ireland according to the Department of Health, Social Services and Public Safety.

The main types of dementia include:

Alzheimer's disease This is the most common cause of dementia. According to Alzheimer's Society, there are more than 520,000 people in the UK with Alzheimer's disease. It is named after a German psychiatrist called Alois Alzheimer, who first noticed the condition in the early 1900s in a 51-year-old female patient called Auguste Deter, who was suffering from short-term memory loss. During her autopsy in 1906, it was discovered that she had shrinkage of the cortex (the largest part of the brain) and abnormal deposits in and around nerve cells.

Proteins that build up in the brain to form structures called plaques and tangles are the cause, as they affect connections between nerve cells, eventually causing them to die.

Alzheimer's disease has two forms, the rare early-onset disease, where symptoms first appear under the age of 65, and the more common late onset Alzheimer's where symptoms appear over this age.

Symptoms: memory loss, difficulty learning new skills or new informa-tion, repeating things, confusion, loss of concentration, depression and irritability.

Vascular dementia This is the second most common type of dementia and according to Alzheimer's Society it affects around 150,000 people in the UK. Vascular dementia is caused by a reduced blood flow to the brain that can be caused by a series of mini-strokes, or by small blood vessels deep in the brain becoming narrowed and hardened (atherosclerosis). Vascular dementia is more common in smokers, those with high blood pressure, Type 2 diabetes, obesity or heart problems. Age is also a strong risk factor.

Symptoms: confusion, problems with concentration, hallucinations, slower thought patterns, memory loss, language problems, depression, anxiety and rapid changes in mood.

Mixed dementia Alzheimer's Society estimates that around 10 per cent of those with dementia have more than one type. Most commonly, people will have a combination of Alzheimer's disease and vascular dementia.

Symptoms: these can vary, depending on the areas of the brain affected. Symptoms could be similar to or the same as symptoms of Alzheimer's disease.

Dementia with Lewy bodies This is estimated to affect around 10 per cent of those with dementia. It is named after Friedrich H. Lewy, a scientist who discovered the condition when researching Parkinson's disease in the early 1900s. Lewy bodies are lumps of protein that develop inside brain cells. Although more research is needed, it is believed that these proteins interfere with chemical messengers in the brain that regulate memory, mood and our ability to learn. Lewy bodies are the cause of several diseases that affect the brain and nervous system, including Parkinson's disease. A person with Parkinson's disease may eventually develop dementia.

Symptoms: fluctuating attention, problems with perception, hallucination, difficulty with balance and movement, disrupted sleep, feelings of being persecuted.

Frontotemporal dementia Also known as Pick's disease, this is a less common form of dementia whereby the two frontal lobes of the brain behind the forehead and the temporal lobes behind the ears are damaged. Brain tissue in the frontal and temporal lobes shrinks. It is often diagnosed in those aged between 45 and 65.

Symptoms: inappropriate behaviour, lack of motivation, cravings for sweet foods, difficulty with speech and difficulty recognizing others.

Getting a diagnosis

If you think your loved one has dementia, it may take some time to persuade him or her to visit the GP. The person may not think anything is wrong, or may blame the symptoms on stress or getting older (the NHS estimates that around 40 per cent of those over 65 will have some form of memory problem). If he or she refuses to visit the GP, then you could talk to the doctor on your own. At least your concerns will be on record.

Getting a diagnosis may take some time. The GP will need to rule out other possible causes of memory loss. She may recommend blood tests to look at iron levels and levels of vitamin B1 and also screen the person for depression, which can cause memory issues. Other conditions that may have similar symptoms to dementia include urinary tract infections and thyroid deficiencies. It's also important to rule out confusion that may be caused by poor sight or hearing. If the tests come back negative, the GP will make a referral to a specialist. This could be a psychiatrist, geriatrician or neurologist. The person with dementia will probably undergo a Mini Mental State Examination (MMSE), which tests memory, thinking and language, and may also be referred for a brain scan.

If the diagnosis is confirmed, the person will be under the care of the local community mental health team – namely psychiatrists, psychologists and community psychiatric nurses. Medication may also be given.

Medication for dementia

There are four types of medication prescribed to treat symptoms of Alzheimer's disease. However, apart from for Alzheimer's, there are no dementia-specific drugs available. The person may also be given other drugs to treat underlying conditions, such as heart disease, a stroke in the case of vascular dementia, or symptoms, such as hallucinations suffered by a person who has dementia with Lewy bodies. A person with vascular dementia may be given drugs to treat high blood pressure, high cholesterol, diabetes or heart problems as these can be linked to the condition. Specialist drugs are only available for people with Alzheimer's disease.

Medication for Alzheimer's disease may slow down the progression of symptoms, but not the disease. They may help to reduce depression, aggression and anxiety, although the drugs will only work for some people. The current four types of medication used to treat Alzheimer's disease include:

- donepezil (Aricept)
- rivastigmine (Exelon)

- galantamine (Reminyl)
- memantine (Ebixa or Axura).

Donepezil, rivastigmine and galantamine are known as cholinesterase inhibitors and work by boosting levels of a chemical messenger called acetylcholine (ACh), which improves communication between the nerve cells. Side effects include vomiting and diarrhoea. These drugs may be beneficial for those with mild to moderate Alzheimer's disease. They are not a cure and the condition is still progressing, but they can treat symptoms in some people. They may not work for everyone.

Memantine is usually prescribed for those with severe Alzheimer's disease, or those with moderate Alzheimer's if cholinesterase inhibitors aren't suitable. It works by regulating activity of glutamate, a chemical messenger involved in brain functions that is released excessively when brain cells are damaged. Side effects can include dizziness, aggression, depression, headaches and sleepiness.

If you have any concerns about any medication prescribed – for example, if you notice any changes in behaviour or side effects – always discuss these immediately with the person's GP or mental health team.

2

What to do when the person is first diagnosed

Even though you might have suspected the person has dementia, the diagnosis could still be a shock. Your parent may be confused and unable to process the news. She may understand the diagnosis, but could be in denial and may refuse any offers of help and support.

You both need some time to come to terms with the diagnosis, but keep talking. Reassure the person. Let her know she isn't alone and get her to talk about it if she wants to. Make it clear you'll be there for her.

But don't wait for too long. It's important for the person to get her affairs in order. Sit down with her and help her plan for the future.

Here's a brief checklist of things to organize as swiftly as possible:

Set up direct debits or standing orders for regular bills As her condition gets worse, she will be more likely to lose her post and may forget to pay bills. Having household bills debited automatically from her account every month will eliminate the risk of having gas or electricity disconnected.

Locate important documents Find out where she keeps other important documents like insurance policies for house and car insurance. If she doesn't object, take these documents home with you and keep a note of any important renewal dates in your diary. Otherwise, put them all in one marked file in a safe place.

File bank statements carefully Keep them in a clearly labelled folder. Again, if she is happy for you to keep hold of these items you can keep track of everything (or arrange online access to accounts). As her condition deteriorates, she will become less able to remember where to put things and items may end up in the most unlikely places.

Get spare house keys cut The person may get locked out of the house, so get a spare set for you and a trusted neighbour.

Encourage the person to make a Lasting Power of Attorney (LPA) as soon as possible This will enable you to make decisions about her health and welfare or her finances when she is no longer able to do so. It needs to be done early on while the person with dementia still has capacity. She won't be able to make a Lasting Power of Attorney if she is considered to lack capacity. This is why it's important to organize this straight away. (See Chapter 3.)

Encourage the person to make or update a will A diagnosis of dementia doesn't mean someone is going to die in the short term, as dementia can take up to around ten years to progress. A person with Alzheimer's disease can live for an average of eight years, or even up to 20 years. However, it's important to make or update a will while the person still has capacity.

Encourage the person to make an Advance Decision This is a legally binding document, which outlines what treatment and end-of-life care a person would like to receive in future.

Obtain third-party authority on the person's bank accounts This means that the person is letting the bank know she would like you to have access to her bank accounts and the ability to manage them in future. You will then have the authority to check her bank balances, transfer funds, make online payments for her and order cheque books on her behalf. You will need to go into the bank with your parent and both of you will need to take identification, including passports and proof of address. For some banks, Lasting Power of Attorney for Property and Finance would also give you this authority, so it may not be necessary, but the situation can vary depending on the bank.

Let the DVLA know about the dementia diagnosis   People have a legal obligation to let the DVLA know they have dementia but may not have to stop driving straight away.

Some of these tasks are outlined in detail in the next chapter.

3

Taking care of the paperwork

It's important to get the person's paperwork in order soon so that everything is taken care of and you can continue to meet his changing needs and wishes in the future.

Setting up a Lasting Power of Attorney

It's recommended that you get this prepared and registered straight away, while the person with dementia still has capacity. If a solicitor thinks someone lacks mental capacity, you might not be able to proceed with the Lasting Power of Attorney, so don't hesitate to start the process. There are two types of Lasting Power of Attorney:

Property and Finance LPA

If the person with dementia appoints you to be his attorney for Property and Finance, this means you can make decisions on matters such as selling his property, investing money on his behalf and paying his bills. You can apply for Lasting Power of Attorney on your own, or the person with dementia can have more than one person acting on his behalf. A solicitor will usually recommend that the person appoints at least two attorneys or, alternatively, one attorney and a replacement attorney. If you have siblings, you might wish to share the responsibility and decisions. It's essential that you trust the other attorneys and feel sure that they have the person's best interests at heart.

With Property and Finance LPA, the person with dementia can delegate decisions to be made on his behalf while he still has capacity. He may choose to pass on decisions to his attorney(s) if he is feeling tired or unwell and doesn't feel able to cope with the burden of making those decisions.

If you are unsure about whether or not the person with dementia still has capacity to make a Lasting Power of Attorney, it's worth seeing a solicitor. The person with dementia must understand what he is signing at that particular moment, and be able to explain to the solicitor if necessary the purpose of what he is doing.

Health and Welfare LPA

Again, the person with dementia will appoint you or you and several other people to be attorneys, to make decisions about his health and well-being. This can include decisions about his medical care and where he lives. It's an essential document to have for the future and you must act with the best of intentions and with the person's wishes in mind. So for instance, if he tells you he doesn't want to go into a care home in future, you have a duty to do all you can to ensure that this doesn't happen, unless it's the only way to keep him safe after all other options have been explored and deemed unsuitable.

Unlike Property and Finance LPA, where the person with dementia can ask the attorney to make decisions for him while he still has capacity, with Health and Welfare LPA the person with dementia must make his own decisions while he still has capacity.

Many people tend to focus on setting up Property and Finance LPA but both types of Lasting Power of Attorney are important. There is no limit to the number of attorneys the person can have and he can choose different attorneys for each type. The roles are very different – some people may be better at making financial decisions than making choices related to health.

There are three different ways of setting up a Lasting Power of Attorney. They are:

Jointly The attorneys have to make decisions together and must all sign paperwork together.

Jointly and Severally Where one or more person(s) can act on behalf of the other attorneys. Many people choose this option. This means that one attorney can sign the paperwork and make decisions without the other attorneys present. This could work well if one of the attorneys lives abroad or frequently works away from home.

Jointly and Jointly and Severally   This means Jointly in respect of some matters and Jointly and Severally in respect of other matters. But you have to be very specific about what matters are going to be Joint and what matters will be Joint and Several.

The person doesn't have to use a solicitor to set up a Lasting Power of Attorney. You can make one online using the Office of the Public Guardian's website: <https://www.gov.uk/government/collections/lasting-power-of-attorney-forms>.

If the person uses a solicitor, once the paperwork has been drawn up and signed, it must be sent to the Office of the Public Guardian, as the Power of Attorney needs to be registered. It takes around six to eight weeks for this to happen.

For more information on making a Lasting Power of Attorney, go to the above link or call the Office of the Public Guardian on 0300 456 0300.

What happens if the person doesn't have mental capacity?

If a solicitor is in any doubt about the person's ability to understand what he is signing and what the Lasting Power of Attorney means, she won't be able to proceed. Sometimes it can be difficult to tell if the person has capacity and the solicitor may seek medical opinions and write to the person's GP. She may ask the GP to act as a Certificate Provider (someone who confirms that the person with dementia understands the nature of the Lasting Power of Attorney).

It's usually in the later stages of dementia that a person has less capacity, and hopefully he won't have left it that long. If he is considered to be lacking capacity, an application to the Court of Protection will need to be made for a 'deputy' to be appointed. This means that the court has jurisdiction to appoint someone to make decisions for the person with dementia. The person is called a deputy and the role is the same as that of an attorney – the difference is that the court, rather than the person with dementia, will appoint the deputy. The process is time-consuming and expensive. It can take up to six months.

Making an Advance Decision

Also known as an Advance Directive, an Advance Decision is a legally binding document, which outlines what treatment and end-of-life care a person would like to receive in future, when he is no longer able to express or communicate what treatment he would like. It's important to prepare an Advance Decision, while the person still has capacity. Examples could be expressing a wish to have his organs donated after he dies or whether or not he would want to be resuscitated if he were to stop breathing in the later stages of his dementia. Another example could be deciding he would not want antibiotics prescribed if he developed pneumonia during the later stages of his dementia. This may sound morbid, but it's important to ensure that the person's wishes are met. The decision must be relevant to the medical circumstances that have arisen and can only be used if the person no longer has capacity.

A person with dementia can write his own Advance Decision but he needs to be clear about his wishes and describe specific scenarios like the examples mentioned. It's worth the person with dementia discussing his Advance Decision with his GP first and if he is still unsure or has further questions, he could discuss them with a solicitor, although he doesn't have to use a solicitor to prepare an Advance Decision. It's sensible to inform his GP that he has made one and make sure his GP has a copy. If he writes his own Advance Decision, it must include the following information:

- his name
- his address
- his date of birth
- the name, address and telephone number of his GP
- the date and his signature.

He should arrange for someone over 18 to sign and witness the document, and let his solicitor have a copy. Incidentally, the laws are different in Northern Ireland. For more information, or for a template of an Advance Decision, visit Alzheimer's Society's website at <https://www.alzheimers.org.uk/site/scripts/documents_info. php?documentID=354>.

Driving with dementia

A diagnosis of dementia doesn't necessarily mean the person has to stop driving immediately. However, he does have a legal obligation to notify the DVLA (in England, Scotland and Wales) or the DVLNI (in Northern Ireland) of his diagnosis immediately. If he doesn't notify the DVLA or DVLNI of any medical conditions that may affect his driving, he could be fined up to £1,000 and could be prosecuted if he is involved in an accident.

To inform the DVLA, he will need to download and complete a form called CG1, a four-page questionnaire from the DVLA's website. If he has been diagnosed with dementia with Lewy bodies, he will need to fill in a B1 form. The form will ask for details of his GP and consultant if he has one, along with the name of any clinics he is attending and details of his medication.

When he downloads the form, he will also receive a medical consent form which, when completed, will give the DVLA authority to write to his GP and arrange for the GP to release any relevant medical information it needs. The DVLA will then assess whether the person with dementia is fit to drive. In some cases, he may be advised to stop driving as a precaution until assessments are carried out. This can take several weeks. If the DVLA decides he is eligible to drive, it will issue a new driving licence for a fixed period, usually of around one to three years, depending on the current stage of the dementia. His condition will usually be reviewed about once a year.

You may want to help your parent fill in the relevant form. He may be angry about his driving being under scrutiny. Remind him he has a legal obligation to do this. If he doesn't, he will be breaking the law. If the DVLA decides it is not safe for him to drive, or you decide he is putting himself at risk by driving, then try to help him get out as much as possible to prevent him getting more frustrated.

You can reach the DVLA on 0300 790 6802 or visit the website at <https://www.gov.uk/dementia-and-driving> or write to them at:

DVLA
Swansea
SA99 1DF

4

Knowing whom you can trust

It's a sad fact that having dementia puts a person at greater risk of being a victim of fraud or financial wrongdoing. Friends or even members of the person's own family can exploit her, as it may be difficult or impossible for her to manage her own affairs. According to a Financial Abuse Review published by Age UK in November 2015, those with dementia or reduced cognitive function are most at risk. The review also revealed that:

- 50 per cent of financial abuse in the UK is by 'adult children', i.e. grown-up sons and daughters;
- approximately 130,000 people aged 65 and over have suffered financial abuse since turning 65, though this is considered to be a conservative estimate.

Another review conducted for Age UK in 2008 showed that 70 per cent of financial abuse is by a family member. A report by King's College London and the National Centre for Social Research published in 2007 revealed that 57,000 people aged 66 and over in the UK had suffered financial abuse by a relative, friend or careworker.

So while you will have your parent's best interests in mind, others may not. If you are managing the person's finances, you may not think she is at risk, but don't rule out the possibility of people taking advantage of her in other ways. I've heard stories of repairmen overcharging and relatives asking the person with dementia to 'write a blank cheque' to pay for some shopping, and then rounding up the amount. I've even heard of relatives going out for dinner, without the person, and then using her debit card to pay for the meal.

Although being a carer can be a stressful task, there is no justification for taking what isn't rightly yours. It's incredible how many people believe they have an 'early inheritance' due because they are caring for the very person who cared for them when they were younger.

If your instincts tell you that someone is guilty of wrongdoing, then don't ignore any nagging doubts. Address the matter at once and take all the necessary steps to protect the person with dementia. Report the matter to the police. Keep her cheque book and debit cards in a safe place. Order her shopping online so that she doesn't need to carry much cash. If you are managing her finances with someone else, or someone else is managing her finances, be extremely wary of anyone who refuses to be open and share information with you. You might think it would never happen in your family. You'd be surprised.

Jane's story

My mother had vascular dementia and lived alone after my father died. My sister insisted on taking care of all Mum's finances and wouldn't let me help. Mum didn't object. When Mum's needs increased and it became apparent that she would need to go into a care home, I asked my sister if we could look at Mum's finances. She refused and became very guarded, so I grew suspicious. I was advised to get third-party authority on Mum's bank accounts, which meant I would be able to look at her bank balances. I found out that my sister had been making substantial and regular monthly withdrawals from Mum's bank account without her consent. I wouldn't have believed it if I hadn't seen it with my own eyes. It turned out my sister was only interested in Mum's money.

If you suspect something, here are some things you can do:

- Speak to the person's bank if you suspect theft from her bank account and explain what you think may have occurred.
- Cancel all debit cards immediately.
- Obtain third-party access on the person's account (see p. 8) so that you can monitor activity.
- If theft has occurred, report the matter to the police and obtain a crime reference number for the bank, which they may require in order to investigate the matter.
- Seek advice urgently. Call the charity Action on Elder Abuse for advice on 080 8808 8141, or alternatively, speak to Age UK's helpline on 0800 169 2081.

If you are concerned about someone abusing a Lasting Power of Attorney, it can be revoked if the person with dementia still has capacity. Contact the Office of the Public Guardian on 0300 456 0300 or by email at <opg.safeguardingunit@publicguardian.gsi.gov.uk> or speak to a solicitor for further advice.

Above all, if something doesn't seem right then it probably isn't. Never ignore your instincts. I know many people who thought it would never happen in their family and now wish they could turn back the clock.

5

Getting help with providing care

You may be concerned about how you will care for the person with dementia. You may not live near the person, may be the only relative or may work full time and have a family. When my mother was first diagnosed and it became apparent she was going to need support, I remember feeling very anxious about how I would be able to meet her needs. The point is that I couldn't provide all of that support alone. You may be in a similar situation. So what can you do?

Friends and family

Encourage friends and family to rally round, and try to draw up a rota of visits/chores. Work together as a team for the benefit of the person with dementia. Communicate regularly about your planned visits and how the person is coping. If you notice any changes in his health, let others know (and of course the person's GP) and keep talking. You'll feel supported and it will also benefit the person with dementia.

You may be wondering what other support is available. There are regional variations and the situation is different in Scotland, Northern Ireland and Wales, but broadly in England, there are three systems:

- The social care system – this is run by the local authority.
- The welfare benefits system – under this system the person with dementia may be entitled to Attendance Allowance.
- The NHS – under this system the person may be eligible for Continuing Care.

So where do you start to search for help?

Wherever you live, start with the social care system, and this means contacting the person's local authority (council) and asking for an assessment of his needs to see if he is eligible for local authority funding. The Care Act 2014 stipulates that the person must have access to good quality information and advice from the first time he contacts the local authority. The person is entitled to an assessment to see if he meets certain eligibility criteria. This is called a Needs Assessment. The criteria for eligibility tend to be restricted to those with high levels of need and therefore it can be difficult to get funding.

If the person qualifies for funding, the care is means-tested; in other words, the person's assets, including his savings and the value of his home, will be considered. He might well qualify for care but may be expected to fully fund it himself. You might then wonder if he would be better off appointing his own home-care agency directly. If you arrange care privately, the local authority would not oversee it and so your rights against that provider are entirely in the terms of the contract that you have with the agency. If the local authority provide that care, they have a statutory duty to ensure the care is meeting the person's needs. If it isn't, the person could use the local authority's complaints system and they would look into what has been going wrong. So it provides some level of protection.

If the person is not considered eligible for financial support from the local authority, the authority should still give him information and advice about what care he needs and how he can go about finding it. For instance, if the local authority think that the person might qualify for NHS support, they should link his assessment to the NHS. To find your local social services department, visit <https://www.gov.uk/help-care-support>.

Attendance Allowance

This is provided by the Department of Work and Pensions (DWP) to those who are 65 and over who require help with personal care. It is not means-tested and is tax-free. There are two levels of financial assistance. A lower rate may apply if the person requires frequent or constant supervision during the day or at night, while a higher rate will apply if he requires help and supervision *throughout* the day and night, or if he is terminally ill. For more information, visit the DWP website at <https://www.gov.uk/attendance-allowance>.

To download an Attendance Allowance claim form from the website, visit <https://www.gov.uk/government/publications/attendance-allowance-claim-form>.

The form will ask about your parent's illness, how long he has been ill, what medication he is taking, treatment received and details of any hospital visits. The DWP may want to contact his GP. It may ask if your parent has any aids at home, such as a stair lift, and you will be asked to describe his current care needs. It's best if you complete the form on behalf of your parent, as the questions are detailed. Get him to sign it and post it for him. If your parent is turned down for Attendance Allowance, he can appeal against the decision. For more information, visit the DWP website.

If your parent does receive Attendance Allowance, he could also obtain extra Pension Credit, Housing Benefit or Council Tax reduction. Speak to the DWP helpline. The amounts will be paid into his bank account directly each month if he obtains financial help.

If your parent is under the age of 65, he may be entitled to help from the Personal Independence Payment and Disability Living Allowance (PIP). This is gradually replacing the Disability Living Allowance and is also tax-free, payable every month. There are two rates, Daily Living Component and Mobility Component. Daily Living is for those who need help with washing and dressing, preparing or eating food and managing medication. Mobility is for those who have trouble moving around and getting out. To qualify, the person must have had problems for at least three months and expect these needs to last for at least nine months. For information, visit <https://www.gov.uk/pip/overview>.

At the time of writing, there is talk of Attendance Allowance being abolished for new claimants, though people currently receiving it should not be affected. The government is debating giving the money to local authorities in order for them to administer the allowance. However, the changes are not expected to affect new claimants until 2018 onwards and this information may be subject to change.

NHS Continuing Healthcare

This is a package of care arranged and funded by the NHS that can be in any setting – in the person's home or in a care home. It is available in England, Wales, Scotland and Northern Ireland, though the details below may be different in Northern Ireland.

If the person is eligible, it is free and is not means-tested. The NHS will pay for services from a community nurse or a specialist therapist and associated social care needs such as personal care and domestic tasks.

Anyone over 18 years of age who is assessed as having a certain level of care needs may be entitled to NHS Continuing Healthcare. The assessment must show that the person has a 'primary health need'. There are four elements that are assessed, as follows:

- nature – the characteristics and type of the person's needs and the effect those needs have on the person;
- complexity – the level of skills required to manage the person's needs;
- intensity – the extent and severity of the person's needs and the support needed to meet them;
- unpredictability – how hard it is to predict a change in the person's needs and risks to the person if his needs are not adequately managed.

For more information on NHS Continuing Healthcare in England, visit <www.nhs.uk/conditions/social-care-and-support-guide/pages/nhs-continuing-care.aspx>.

For information about care in Scotland, visit <www.isdscotland.org/Health-Topics/Health-and-Social-Community-Care/NHS-Continuing-Care/>.

For information about NHS Continuing Care in Wales, visit <www.wales.nhs.uk/continuingnhshealthcare>.

For information about NHS Continuing Care in Northern Ireland, contact your local health and social care trust. Find the nearest one by visiting <www.nidirect.gov.uk/health-and-social-care-trusts>.

Carer's Allowance

You might also be entitled to a Carer's Allowance. This is paid to those who provide regular and substantial support and, at the time of writing, you may be entitled to it if:

- you look after someone who gets qualifying disability benefit;
- you are caring for someone for at least 35 hours a week;
- you are aged 16 or over;
- you are not in full-time education;
- you earn £110 a week (after deductions) or less;
- you satisfy UK presence and residence conditions.

For more information, visit <www.carers.org> or call the Carers UK Advice Line on 0808 808 7777.

Seeking advice

This may all sound overwhelming, but advice is available. Age UK has a free Advice Line on 0800 169 2081. It also has local branches and you can find your nearest one by visiting the Age UK website at <www.ageuk.org.uk/no-one/we-provide-advice/> and entering your location.

The Carers UK website can also provide help and support. You can call the Carers UK advice line on 0808 808 7777 or email <advice@carersuk.org>.

Or contact the Citizens Advice Bureau or visit the website at <https://www.citizensadvice.org.uk>, or call 03444 111 444 in England, or in Wales call 03444 77 20 20.

Free help is also available from Alzheimer's Society's National Dementia Helpline on 0300 222 11 22.

Support for you

As a carer, you have a legal right to ask your employer for flexible working hours. It doesn't matter what level of care you are providing for a loved one. It can be visiting him for two hours on a weekend to make sure he is OK, or visiting him every day. If you are providing care, then you can request flexibility.

Your employer is not obliged to agree but has to consider your request. If it is refused, you must be given a specific reason.

Small things may help. I would sometimes leave work early to take Mum to an appointment, or I'd work from home. So long as I met my deadlines, my employer raised no objections. If you have a good relationship with your boss then talk to her, explain the situation and you may find she is supportive.

You also have the right to take a reasonable amount of time off in the event of an emergency. It's up to your employer to decide whether this is paid or unpaid.

In addition, you are entitled to an assessment of your own needs by the local authority, even if you are not a full-time carer. If you are not entitled to Carer's Allowance, the assessment may still result in you being offered support to enable you to continue to care for the person, such as a respite break or arranging for the person with dementia to go to a day centre one day a week to give you a break, or perhaps even help with travel arrangements if you live a long way from the person.

Finally, it's worth noting that there may be some regional variations on available support. Contact your local authority (council) for more details of help in your area.

6

Making the person safe at home

If your parent lives alone, it's going to take some foresight and planning to ensure she remains safe in her own home. She may still be fairly independent at the moment but make no mistake – her needs will increase over time and she may already need help with certain tasks. At this point, you may want to consider:

Current challenges Identify what the person currently needs help with, what help could be provided, and how that help will be provided.

Support available Even if you are in a position where you are able to become a full-time carer, you will still need help as there will come a time when the person with dementia can't be left alone. Don't try and do it all on your own. Rikki Lorenti, an Admiral Nurse from SweetTree Home Care Services, recommends the following:

- seeking as much information as possible about the health of the person from the Memory Clinic;
- making sure the rest of your family are aware of the situation so that the burden of caring for the person can be shared;
- seeking advice from a Dementia Care Adviser or your local Alzheimer's Society;
- finding someone to talk to, such as a local carers' support group;
- finding out if there is a local Admiral Nurse in your area – Admiral Nurses were developed in the late 1980s to provide support, guidance and knowledge for families coping with dementia. They can recommend strategies and suggest practical ways of coping. To find out if there is an Admiral Nurse in your area, visit <https://www.dementiauk.org/>.

Where is the person now?

In the early stages of dementia, it may be safe for the person to go out on her own and live reasonably independently. As her needs increase, she may go out without a house key, leave the front door open or wander off. Identifying these possible scenarios now may help to prevent them.

Current challenges

Some extra support may be sufficient in the early days of the person's diagnosis. It might be a case of someone coming in to do the housework once a week, or taking her to the shops every couple of days.

You could ask your parent what help she needs but you may not get a straight answer and she may not like you implying she can't cope on her own. She may tell you she doesn't need help. Rely on your instincts and take note of what you see. Don't rely solely on the information the person is giving you – she may genuinely think there is nothing wrong. Or she may be in denial.

Ginny's story
One of the biggest challenges was knowing when to take control of aspects of Mum's life. When to take the car keys away. When to start doing the washing. When to buy her food. When to switch the oven off at the mains. Day after day, all these questions. Each one tinged with sadness.

It's difficult to know when to take charge but you have to be strong and go with your instincts. Even if the person thinks she doesn't need help, if the evidence tells you otherwise then you have a duty to do your best for her. As the dementia progresses, you will become the parent and she will become the child. You will become an expert at knowing what is best for her, in the same way that a parent knows what is best for a child.

My mother began to lose weight in the early stages of her diagnosis. When we discussed my concerns, she insisted that she was eating three balanced meals every day, but her fridge and cupboards told a different story. I could only find chocolate and a few slices of out-of-date ham in her fridge, and her cupboards were full of tinned foods three years out of date. I arranged for her to have Meals on Wheels through social services, so that she had hot, nutritious meals every day. Her weight increased and her health improved.

Overcoming objections

You may meet with resistance when offering help but if you feel there is a genuine need for it then be patient and gently persevere. At first, my mum didn't want Meals on Wheels and complained about the food. I persuaded her to be patient and keep trying them. I said we would cancel the meals at the end of the week if she still didn't like them. After a few days, she realized that each meal came with a pudding, and the pudding won her over! She grew to like the meals and I felt happier knowing that someone was delivering her healthy food every day, as it meant she would also be checked up on at the same time.

Convincing the person that she needs help may become a negotiation. Other times, you have to just go with your instincts and do what you feel is right for the person and hope she gets used to it. This may sound heavy-handed, but over time you will know best. She may not always agree with you. Stand your ground.

Be observant

There are many examples of where the person with dementia will need help, so keep observing her, but do it discreetly so that she doesn't get defensive. If the laundry is piling up, then get someone in to help with washing, or load up the washing machine when you visit. Incidentally, the person with dementia may have forgotten how to use the washing machine. Or she may not even notice her clothes are dirty.

Domestic appliances may become a source of confusion. You may think that written instructions are an obvious solution but there is no guarantee that she will be able to process what you've written. If a washing machine or microwave breaks down and needs replacing, she may struggle to learn how to use a new one and you may need a careworker to come in and take care of some domestic tasks.

What needs doing?

When you visit, look around the house. Is she changing her bedding regularly? Is the house messy or dirty? Is the garden becoming overgrown? Is she still able to do some of the things she liked to do before? My mother used to enjoy going out for a walk in her village. She knew the locals and they looked out for her. Eventually, she was unable to find her way back home and it became impossible for her to go out on her own. She lost confidence and stopped going out altogether. Each time I visited, I made sure we went out for lunch or to the shops, so that she was still getting some fresh air and stimulation. Think about what the person with dementia would like to do and what help she will need to keep doing what she enjoys. Then think about who can provide that help or support, be it a neighbour, a relative or a paid careworker.

A safe environment

Ask yourself whether the home is a safe environment for the person with dementia. Will she remember to turn the oven off, lock up at night and turn off the TV when she goes to bed? You may want to spend the night to see how she is managing with these tasks – let her go through her bedtime routine of shutting everything off and see if she can do it, unprompted by you. If not, you may need someone to come in and help.

Is it safe for her to cook her own meals? My mother hated cooking, so it was no biggie for me to disconnect her oven. You may need to turn the oven off at the mains, or arrange for the person to have a convection oven that turns itself off when food is cooked, though you've still got the challenge of her learning how to use it.

There are companies who can install monitors in the house and provide pendant alarms and GPS navigation, which will track the person when she leaves the house. This may sound drastic and may not be needed at this stage, but it's important to keep thinking ahead. Talk to Adult Social Care in your local social services department in the first instance.

Is it safe for the person to load the washing machine when she is at home alone? Consider disconnecting it and taking her laundry home with you. Disconnect any portable fires if you are concerned and set her central heating so that the house is warm and the heating automatically goes off.

Risk of falls

Mobility may be an issue and this could increase the risk of falls. The person's home can be adapted to be made safer. It's worth contacting the GP, social services or the local Alzheimer's Society office if you have one. The GP or social services may be able to arrange for an occupational therapist to come in and recommend changes or adaptations that may be provided by social services. This could include items like a handrail for the stairs, a bath seat, a raised toilet seat, a shower stool and mobility aids like a walking frame. Resources vary depending on where you live, and you may have to wait for this service, so if you feel it's time-sensitive, then you can buy a variety of walking aids online. A commode might be a good idea if the person with dementia is prone to waking at night, as it will mean she doesn't have to move very far to reach the toilet. Getting a small nightlight for the person with dementia may also be a good idea, so that she is less likely to fall over or get confused in the dark.

Alzheimer's Society has a good factsheet on its website about how to keep the person safe at home, and it recommends the following to help prevent the risk of falls:

- Check the house for potential hazards such as rugs, worn or loose carpets, furniture in awkward places and objects (e.g. flexes) on the floor.
- Encourage the person to exercise – this can improve strength and balance.
- Keep the person's feet healthy – foot pain and long toenails can increase risk of falls. A regular visit to a podiatrist or chiropodist is a good idea. The person's GP surgery may be able to recommend a local chiropodist.
- Check her eyesight – make sure the person has regular eye tests. Make sure her home is well lit.
- Keep objects within easy reach – anything used regularly should be easy for the person to get to.

Alzheimer's Society has some useful information on its website about making the person's house safe. Visit <https://www.alzheimers.org.uk/site/scripts/documents_info.php?documentID=3113>.

Medication

Is it safe for the person to take her medication unsupervised and will she remember to take it? In the early days of her diagnosis, my mum needed a daily phone call to remind her to take her tablets (though I stayed on the phone while she took them). She knew which ones to take and just needed reminding. As she got worse, the tablets had to be split up into days of the week using a medical dosset box (a box divided into sections for different days of the week, available online or from pharmacies). I filled the box up once a week. This worked for a time. Then one day I went to visit her and found all of the tablets from the entire dosset box spread out on the dining room table. I realized that Mum could no longer take her tablets unsupervised. I bought a portable safe to store the tablets, and arranged for a home careworker to administer them. Mum only ever took them under supervision from that point on. If in doubt, lock medication away.

Food sources

If your parent isn't eating properly, speak to social services about arranging for Meals on Wheels to be delivered. The person may have to pay for it but it's not expensive. She will receive meals every day, delivered by a local volunteer. And you have the added bonus of someone checking up on her.

Alarms and key safes

When you speak to social services, it's also worth enquiring about a pendant alarm or key safe. A key safe is a small box with a unique PIN code on the front that can be installed on the wall outside the person's house to store a spare key. Social services can arrange this and may also arrange for someone to come and install it, though you may need to pay. My mum had one installed (against her wishes) but it proved invaluable on occasions when she locked herself out or a careworker needed to gain access when she couldn't hear the front door. You can also buy them online.

A pendant alarm (also known as a personal alarm) is another useful item that the person wears around her neck, like a necklace. If she has a fall when she is alone, it means she can press a button on the pendant and call for help 24 hours a day, seven days a week (the calls go through to an emergency response unit). Admittedly, this wasn't ideal for my mother as she would forget to wear it – so it does have its limitations but may be of some use in the earlier stages of dementia. If you think your parent might wear it then it may be worth getting one. They also come as wristbands. Ask social services about obtaining one, or you can buy one direct from Age UK by calling 0800 028 8782 or visiting <www.ageuk.org.uk/products/mobility-and-independence-at-home/personal-alarms/>.

Simple devices

'Assistive technology' is the term given to products (or the process of selecting suitable products) designed for those with disabilities or dementia. The items are deliberately easy to use and can help in many ways. They include items like simple phones and TV remote controls, with fewer buttons. There are many companies who sell these products online.

So how can they help? My mother began to confuse the TV remote control with her phone, as they were roughly the same size and shape. I bought her a simple Doro phone (a phone made deliberately simple, aimed at older people) containing only numbers for dialling and no other confusing buttons. I replaced her remote control with a simple remote with few buttons. I also bought her an old-fashioned radio similar to one she'd had years before – it could be turned on and off with the press of just one button.

These small changes may not sound significant, but to a person with dementia, they could make a big difference to her quality of life.

Frequency of visits

Regular visits from you or other relatives or careworkers are important, as they will not only help keep the person safe but also keep her mentally stimulated, which can improve her mood and help slow down the symptoms of dementia. But it may be hard to visit frequently if you work full time and don't live locally. My mother lived more than an hour away. I used to visit every weekend and occasionally one day in the week. This was the best I could manage given the demands of my busy job. But here's the important point:

The best I could manage wasn't enough for her.

That didn't mean I wasn't doing my best for Mum. It just meant that what I could realistically do for her and what she needed didn't match. My daily phone calls weren't enough, so clearly I wasn't going to be able to do it all on my own.

I knew I needed help with caring for Mum, so I found it. I spoke to Age UK, who provided a cleaner who went in once a week for two hours. As Mum's needs increased, I arranged for the cleaner to go in more frequently. I also arranged for careworkers to go in and prompt Mum to take her tablets. Later on, it became apparent that Mum needed help getting washed and dressed in the mornings, so I arranged for a careworker to go in and get her out of bed, get her washed and make her breakfast.

Finally, I also arranged for a gardener to look after the garden that she enjoyed looking at but could no longer manage. The gardener later doubled as an odd-job man and a good friend who kept an eye on Mum. If anything needed repairing, he could usually fix it and I knew I could count on him to be efficient and reliable. The more support you can enlist, the better.

If you have relatives willing to help out, then by all means accept that help but make sure you can rely on their support. If they let you down more than once then rule them out of the caring package. Caring for a person with dementia can provide many unpredictable challenges – you can't afford for others to be unpredictable as well.

7

Coping with challenging behaviour

For many years your parent cared for you, and now you probably feel like the parent. You may be mourning for the loss of someone you found dependable, a person you turned to for help and advice many times. Now he may seem lost and even childlike. At the same time, you're still dealing with the practical challenges of looking after him in the present and worrying about what may happen in the future.

Dementia affects the brain so the person may suffer from frequent mood swings. One minute he may be happy, the next he may be shouting, angry or tearful. These moments may be brief – my mother would cry one minute and then laugh at something funny on TV the next. While I was still trying to establish the cause of the tears, she had already moved on.

Anger may be an issue. If the person becomes angry, there could be many reasons:

Pain The person may be unable to express himself or describe what is wrong, so shouting could be a way to defend himself or try to let you know he is in pain. Look for any giveaway signs such as a change in his walking pattern, or he may be holding his head or stomach. You can ask if he is in pain and he may say yes, but he may not be able to explain where the pain is. General analgesia (medication for mild to moderate pain) may help if his GP is happy to prescribe it. (If pain persists, take him back to the doctor.) Other signs of pain may include grimacing, a change in body language, such as tensing up, or being pale or sweaty, which can indicate a high temperature.

Thirst or hunger Has he had enough to eat or drink? Have his eating habits changed recently? Lack of hydration can lead to increased confusion so make sure he has had something to drink.

A urinary tract infection This can also cause increased confusion so it's important to take him to the GP.

Boredom If the person used to be more active, or has recently had to give up driving, for example, he may lack stimulation and this can lead to anger and frustration. Regular social contact with others is important, so try to avoid long periods where the person is sitting in front of the TV with no one to talk to. He could join a social group, or perhaps friends can visit more often to break up his day.

Lack of stimulation As his carer, you are doing your best for the person but you could be doing too much. Get him to help out with a few domestic tasks that will give him a sense of purpose. The more he can do for himself, the better.

Sundowning This is a term that refers to a sudden change of mood that usually affects a person with mid- or late-stage dementia. It tends to occur late in the afternoon or early evening when the sun goes down. Some people believe it is caused by chemical changes in the brain but experts aren't sure of the exact cause. It might be because the person is tired, or bored from sitting around all day. According to one study in *Clinical Geriatrics*, those who had more light late in the day were less agitated. Keeping a room well lit may help. Distraction techniques or activities to stimulate the person may also be useful.

Fear or anxiety Is there a pattern to the mood swings? Do they occur at roughly the same time? My mother would get angry at 4 p.m. This coincided with the time I would normally have to leave. If you can establish whether there is a pattern to this behaviour, then you may be able to address the situation. In my mum's case, it was probably anxiety about being on her own. Reassuring the person that another relative or friend will be in to see him might do the trick.

Being contradicted A person with dementia will need to work much harder than you to keep up with a conversation and formulate a response to questions. This might be exhausting. So imagine how he might feel if he's worked hard to tell you something, and you contradict what he's said. If he is describing a previous experience that you shared with him, and he gets the date or location wrong, don't point this out. Let him remember it the way he wants to. Contradicting him will only undermine his confidence and could make him angry.

Unreasonable behaviour

There may be many times when you feel that the person with dementia is being unreasonable. On a bad day, my mother would throw things or make nasty personal remarks. It took me a while to realize her comments weren't personal. The person with dementia can't change his behaviour and he can't be reasoned with. If a person becomes angry, or can't remember what you said five minutes ago, it's not his fault.

Janice's story
As the dementia took hold, my mum would get very angry. She started to throw things and hit out at my sister and me if we upset her. She was often aggressive. She withdrew into herself. We joined a local dementia group and with their help we got Mum into a day centre three days a week. This was a great help. Music calmed Mum down. She loved music and dancing. Sometimes, however bad it gets, they will laugh with you and you will cry with them. Just let them know you still love them. Hold hands. Give them a hug, but it will have to be on a good day as affection is not always welcome. You will need great patience.

If the person is being aggressive or angry, experts generally advise taking a step back. Admiral Nurse Rikki Lorenti has this advice for coping with anger:

- Don't get into a confrontation – if the environment and risk level is low then go and do something else and come back.
- Remember aggression may be related to frustration – try to find out what is causing the frustration, such as being disorientated or struggling to complete a task.
- Offer guidance to the person if he is trying to do something, but try to allow him control over completing the task.
- Sit near the person and hold on to his hand if he is happy for you to do so.

Rikki has this advice for trying to combat depression, which can manifest itself during the early days of dementia:

- Try to make life as normal as possible and encourage him to keep up hobbies and interests as much as he can.
- Focus on what he can do, rather than what he can't do.
- If mood becomes an issue then discuss this with his GP or the Memory Clinic to consider short-term medication.
- Be aware that insecurity will become more evident as the dementia progresses – a combination of poor recognition, disorientation and the need for reassurance will become more apparent.

Dealing with bereavement

A person with dementia may forget that a loved one has died, and may ask for him or her. When my mother first asked why my father hadn't come home from work, I explained that he died five years ago. I didn't know any better at the time. Mum was not only incredibly distressed about losing her husband of 50 years but also very concerned that she would forget losing him. I felt terrible as I listened to her grieve all over again, as though he had died yesterday. Now if she asks after him or anyone else who has passed away, I will distract or deflect the question by saying: 'Dad is normally at work at this time' and then offer her a cup of tea. The distraction works and she will talk about something else. If a person keeps referring to a dead relative, reassurance may be needed. He may be searching for the familiarity and safety that the person represented.

8

Other unexpected symptoms

You want to do your best for the person with dementia, and you'll do all you can to make her happy. But sometimes ideas that are meant to be a treat or a kind gesture can backfire. When my mum seemed depressed in the early stages of her dementia, I arranged for us to go to a health spa together. She liked beauty treatments, so I booked her a pedicure. But what she would have enjoyed a number of years ago became quite stressful. She didn't like the therapist 'pulling' her feet around and became distressed. The health spa environment unsettled her. Even though it was a luxury resort, she found it unsettling that people walked around in dressing gowns. 'This reminds me of a hospital,' she told me through gritted teeth. We came home a day early.

Leaving the familiar environment of the person's home over-night can be stressful for her. Think carefully before you plan holidays that may cause confusion. Start with a short break at first and see how the person responds before booking a longer break. Everyone is unique but a sudden change in environment or routine may be too much.

Change in appearance

You may have noticed that the person with dementia is not taking much pride in her appearance. This could be because she finds it difficult to wash and dress, or she may simply be less motivated to get washed and dressed or change her clothes properly. This can be a shock when you first notice it, especially if the person was known for taking pride in her appearance.

You may need to help her get washed and dressed or encourage her to take a shower. A shower stool may be a good solution if the person is nervous about slipping over, but it could simply be that she can't see the point in getting washed and dressed.

Julie's story

My mother Angela used to take real pride in how she looked and was quite glamorous in her younger days. But as the dementia took hold, I noticed that she started wearing clothes with food stains on them, and didn't seem bothered when I pointed them out. As time went on, she actually started to smell and I found it very hard to say anything. I arranged for carers to come in and provide personal care but she would insist that she didn't want or need a wash. Some days she'll be more accommodating, other days she isn't interested in changing out of her night clothes.

If you are struggling to persuade the person to get washed and dressed, think about how essential it is at that moment. If she is staying in most of the day then sitting around in her nightwear won't be a big deal and a quick wash may be less stressful for her.

If you are helping the person with personal hygiene, try to make her feel at ease. If she needs to remove her clothes and wash, she may feel violated, even by you. How much help does she really need? If she is in the early or mid stages of dementia, she may be able to manage and may just need a few prompts. Choose clothes that are easy to pull on or take off. Avoid fiddly zips or tops that need to be pulled over the head. Cardigans will be easier to put on than roll-neck jumpers. Tracksuit bottoms or trousers with an elasticated waistband will be easier to put on and remove than jeans or buttoned trousers.

When helping with personal care, try the following:

- Give the person space – allow extra time to help her get washed and dressed if you are taking her out.
- Use distraction techniques – if you are helping her with washing or toileting, do what you can to help while distracting her with a conversation about a topic she likes. A careworker once told me a colleague of hers would tell a resident that she was going for a spa treatment. She would then give her a foot massage with oils afterwards.
- Put yourself in the person's shoes – as a carer, it's easy to focus on the task that needs to be done and not think about the impact it's having on the person with dementia. Imagine how strange it would feel to have someone washing or dressing you.
- Encourage her to be independent – whatever she can still do for

herself, let her do it, without trying to take over and pointing out that she is doing it wrong.

Dementia and sight

Another important consideration when caring for a person with dementia is that her sight can be affected. You may think we see with our eyes, but the brain has to interpret what we see. It is estimated that up to 60 per cent of those with dementia have trouble with impaired vision, and those with dementia with Lewy bodies can hallucinate. If your parent seems lost in a familiar environment, or appears to be struggling to see things, arrange for her to have an eye test and rule out sight problems. If her sight is OK, she may be struggling to identify specific objects or persons, or be receiving distorted information from the brain about what's in front of her.

This could lead to the person becoming more withdrawn, having falls or growing more confused. Colours and patterns can cause confusion. Choose contrasting colours when trying to make certain objects stand out. A red toilet seat on a white basin will help the person sit on the toilet properly, or a blue plate on a white tablecloth will help her identify that food is in front of her. Removing patterned rugs from the floor is a good idea, as the person may view them as obstacles.

Tracy's story
My father had dementia with Lewy bodies, and not only did he suffer from hallucinations from time to time but he also had a problem with the floor tiles in his bathroom. He was confused by the black and white square tiles, and thought the black tiles were holes in the floor. He was terrified of falling through them and tried not to step on them. In the end, we replaced the tiles with a plain floor.

A person with dementia may also think that people or animals on TV are in the same room. You can imagine how distressing this must be, so try to avoid having anything too graphic or violent on television as it could cause unnecessary upset. In some cases, this could be side effects of medication so speak to the GP if you are concerned.

June's story

My mother, who had vascular dementia, phoned me one evening and said there were people in her house who wouldn't leave. I assumed she meant the carers, as she often refused to let them in and didn't like them coming over. But I became concerned when she mentioned there were several people in the house. Then she told me they were standing around drinking and had ignored her requests to leave. I asked her to put them on the phone to me and she replied: 'I can't get their attention.' I could hear some background noise and realized it was the TV. She had confused TV characters with real people.

9

Appointing a home-care agency

As the person's needs increase, you will need to explore various care options to make sure he is receiving the help and support he needs at home. A home careworker could be a good solution and there are several different models:

Direct service This is where the regulated home-care organization employs its own staff and is contracted by you or your parent to provide a home-care service. This could include calling three times a day for one hour to help with getting up, washing and dressing, breakfast and taking medication.

Introductory or employment agency The home-care agency introduces a careworker to you, and you or your parent will then employ that person to carry out tasks. This is a model commonly used for live-in care. Whether these agencies are regulated depends on the regulatory regime of the UK nation concerned. In England, they are not able to register with the Care Quality Commission (CQC).

Personal assistant This is where your parent would recruit and employ a careworker, who would be unregulated. Your parent would be responsible for the personal assistant's tax and national insurance, and would need to provide them with a contract of employment and pay slips. Such an employee would also need to be paid at least the National Living Wage (£7.20 per hour at the time of writing) and would be entitled to benefits like paid holiday and statutory sick pay. It's realistic to expect that the admin tasks linked to this situation would probably fall on your shoulders, so this may not be the best solution.

If you use a direct service, the careworker is employed by the agency, which means they are responsible for paying the careworker and deducting tax, and your parent pays the agency. Home-care agencies are slightly more expensive than a private careworker as you pay their commission as well as the employee's fee, but the service is flexible. Home care can be a few hours a week or much more substantial. It may be appropriate to have a careworker who comes in twice a day to get your parent up and dressed and put him to bed, or three times a day if he needs help with food and domestic tasks like shopping and household duties. You can choose the level of care. An agency will also send a replacement careworker if your parent's regular careworker is ill or on holiday. However, consistency of care is very important when caring for a person with dementia. The more familiar the careworker, the more comfortable the person will feel about having him or her in the house. However, careworkers are obviously entitled to breaks, holidays and sick leave so, in practice, home-care organizations would build a small team of people who are familiar with the person, rather than relying solely on one individual. Even with a live-in careworker, more than one person would be needed to provide care so the careworker can have proper breaks.

What services are provided?

Services provided by a home-care agency may include basic domestic and personal tasks, such as washing, bathing and dressing, and help around the home, such as doing laundry and shopping. However, organizations vary in what they offer – some don't do domestic tasks other than those linked to home care, and some have a domestic arm that is different from home-care services so that it is contracted separately. Some combine home care and domestic services and allow their workers to do both, if it is written into the care plan.

Choosing the right care

Not all home-care agencies have staff trained to deal with a person with dementia. They might be caring for a person with learning disabilities in the morning and then caring for a person with dementia in the afternoon. Finding an agency with dementia-trained staff is a good idea. Ideally, you would need a home-care agency that specializes in dementia. Ask the care manager about the background and experience of the staff and ask for references. Ask to speak to another client who receives care from the agency. It's also worth taking a look at the Care Quality Commission's website, which inspects the service provided and has reports on home-care agencies that rate them in five categories – including whether the CQC felt the agency provides a service that is safe, effective, caring, responsive and well led. Visit the website at <www.cqc.org.uk> and then enter the name of the agency. Care regulators in Scotland are at <www.scswis.com>; for Wales visit <http://cssiw.org.uk>; and for Northern Ireland <www.rqia.org.uk>.

Always meet the manager of the agency and the person who will be caring for your parent. Questions to ask as recommended by the United Kingdom Homecare Association include:

- Can they provide the care needed?
- Have they cared for someone in a similar situation to your parent?
- Do they obtain references from careworkers' previous employers?
- Do all of the careworkers undergo a criminal record disclosure from the Disclosure and Barring Service (in England and Wales) or Disclosure Scotland (in Scotland) or Access NI (in Northern Ireland)?
- What happens if the regular carer is off sick or on holiday?
- Can you contact the agency outside of office hours in an emergency?

If you think your parent simply requires some domestic help at this stage rather than personal care, you may wish to speak to Age UK, who can provide a cleaner for a reasonable hourly rate who will usually also do some shopping. Visit <www.ageuk.org.uk> for more information.

If you use a home-care agency, check that the agency is registered with the United Kingdom Homecare Association (UKHCA), a professional association for home-care providers, whose members agree to comply with a Code of Practice. The UKHCA has a facility to search for a care agency in your parent's area. Visit <www.ukhca.co.uk/findcare/> and enter the postcode.

10

Looking after yourself

Whether you are the main carer or you have a careworker coming in, it's unrealistic to expect to cope with all the emotional and physical demands of caring for the person alone. As the dementia progresses, the person's needs will increase and you may find the situation emotionally more challenging.

Taking care of your own health can often take a back seat. As you focus your energy on making sure your parent is safe and well, your stress levels may increase. And you won't be alone. According to Alzheimer's Society, nine in ten carers for people with dementia experience stress or anxiety several times a week.

Don't neglect your own physical and mental well-being. Having some time to yourself, even if it's just once or twice a week, will make a huge difference to your mental state. If you are no longer mentally and physically healthy, you won't be able to care for your parent.

Regular exercise can make a huge difference to your physical well-being and mental health. The mental health charity Mind recommends regular exercise for reducing symptoms of mild to moderate depression, and the chemicals released during exercise are known to generate a feeling of well-being. A brisk walk or a run offers you a chance to switch off. Or it might be an opportunity to clear your head or solve problems. I found that running really helped with my mental well-being and went on to run a marathon and raise funds for Alzheimer's Society. I felt I was doing some good and taking back control. Without exercise, I honestly don't think I would have coped with taking care of Mum.

Long-term benefits

Experts also believe that regular cardiovascular exercise, like running, cycling, swimming or anything that gets you moderately out of breath, will help to reduce your own risk of developing dementia. According to Alzheimer's Society, of all the lifestyle changes that have been studied, taking regular physical exercise appears to be one of the best things that you can do to reduce your risk of getting dementia. Several prospective studies have looked at middle-aged people and the effects of physical exercise on their thinking in memory and later life. Combining the results of 11 studies shows that regular exercise can significantly reduce the risk of developing dementia by about 30 per cent. For Alzheimer's disease specifically, the risk was reduced by 45 per cent. Regular exercise, three to four times per week, will boost your mood and make you healthier. You'll also sleep better.

Ginny's story
The tiredness and constant anxiety I felt when looking after my mum were significant, but running has always helped me on many levels. It obviously helps keep me fit and slim but it has always been my way to cope with stress and depression. It was a great outlet when I was caring for my mother.

Keep talking

On an emotional level, it's important to find someone to talk to when you need to unload. Find a friend or relative who understands what you are going through. And if no one understands, then talk to Alzheimer's Society or Age UK's helpline team.

Caring for a parent or loved one with dementia takes great strength and courage. You will need to make decisions on his behalf, and you may be grieving for the person he used to be. It's hugely important to deal with any emotional issues you may be facing. If you feel overwhelmed or depressed, don't bottle things up. Talk to your GP and ask to be referred for counselling if you feel it would help.

Encourage your parent to talk about how he is feeling too. While you may be experiencing feelings of grief, he may also be mourning the loss of his independence. It's easy to focus on providing care, but give the person a chance to talk to you. He may also need counselling. Talk to his GP if you suspect this is the case.

11

When the person can no longer live alone

Dementia is a progressive disease and there will come a time when it is no longer safe or practical for the person be alone. You may have already accepted that this is inevitable, and you may already be considering the best next step.

The person with dementia may not be receptive to the idea of moving out and into a care home or living with you or another family member, or may be refusing a live-in careworker. And as a result, you may have had to postpone your plans. However, it could be one unfortunate situation that forces your hand.

Sue's story
My mother had refused to go into a care home even though it wasn't safe for her to live alone any more. She kept telling me that she wasn't a child. I respected her wishes until one day I realized she wasn't safe on her own. One night she locked herself out in the winter at 10 p.m. without a coat. She didn't know what she was doing or where she was going. She couldn't remember where she lived. At that point, I realized that having carers going in daily wasn't enough. When the carers went home, there was no telling what would happen.

It may take something like a specific event or a fall for you to conclude the person can't be alone. Or she may be in hospital as a result of a fall or an infection and you may know she can't return home until she has consistent care.

If she is in hospital, the person should receive an assessment from the local authority that looks at her continuing NHS needs and whether she will have reablement or social care needs when she leaves. Reablement means she would normally receive free care for a period of six weeks when she returns home, such as being prompted to take medication. She may be able to go into a respite home while she recovers.

There will come a time when what your parent wants and what is best for her are two different things. If you want her to go into a care home, your hands may be tied. If your parent has made an Advance Decision that clearly states she does not want to go into a care home, then you do have a duty to act in accordance with her wishes and do your very best to keep her out of one until it is deemed the only safe option.

You may have considered these options:

- a live-in careworker
- sheltered housing or sheltered accommodation
- the person coming to live with you
- a residential care home
- a nursing home.

Live-in care

A live-in careworker may be an option, being with the person most of the time, usually on a rota basis over a weekly, fortnightly or even six-weekly basis, to comply with working-time rules for breaks. The UKHCA is keen to emphasize that the right support will enable people to stay at home and be safe, and stresses that it's no longer automatic that a person should have to go into a care home. This is why it's important to seek advice from everyone involved in the care of your parent. For more information on live-in care, visit <http://stayinmyhome.co.uk>.

Sheltered accommodation

There are two types – sheltered accommodation and extra-care sheltered accommodation. A sheltered housing facility will provide 24-hour support from a warden on site, or via a phone-line support. With extra-care sheltered accommodation there may be additional facilities, such as a communal café or a care scheme that the person would have the option of buying into.

There are different models of sheltered housing as you can either become a tenant of a sheltered housing scheme (talk to the local authority) or buy your own property. More often these days, private companies provide sheltered accommodation. Sheltered accommodation tends to be more suitable for those who can't cope with the size of a large house and garden, who aren't managing household tasks easily and are struggling with stairs. Perhaps they also need occasional help and support and want to be nearer their family.

For a person with dementia, sheltered accommodation may only be a short-term solution, as her needs will increase. If she is already receiving help at home and struggling to cope when the carers go home, then this is unlikely to be a safe option unless there is another person living with her, such as a partner, who is able to help with her care.

Moving the person in with you

It's easy to feel that you should be the one to take care of the person but in reality this may not be practical. Not everyone has the patience or skill to be a full-time carer.

My mother stayed with me on occasions and it was very hard. Some days, it could be rewarding if she was feeling happy. When she had a bad day she could be aggressive and verbally abusive. I would feel resentful towards her and it felt like an emotional roller-coaster. I admit there were many times when my friends were going to social events that I had no time for and I would think: 'I didn't sign up for this.'

When a person has dementia, night and day can become blurred, and she may wake frequently, which means your sleep will also be affected. She may struggle to adjust to the new environment. She may be frustrated by her lack of independence, and that frustration will tend to be directed at her nearest and dearest.

Emotional issues

If you're caring for a parent with dementia, and you've had a troubled relationship in the past, then it's important to try and address any issues that may cause resentment now. To be a good carer, you need to keep your emotions in check. If you have a grudge about the past, it will be hard for you to care for the person without feeling resentful. Deal with any issues now. It may not be realistic to expect the person with dementia to resolve past issues with you, so speak to your GP, who may be able to arrange counselling to help you work through these issues. If you are still struggling with raw memories, then you could hire a careworker to provide part-time assistance to give you a break. Or you may feel that you can't provide the care yourself. If you can't do it then start putting steps in place to make sure the person has adequate care.

If you do want to care for her, remember that the nature and extent of the care will grow. In the early stages, you might only need to do domestic chores, prepare meals and prompt medication. As things change, you'll need to be comfortable with personal care, including washing, bathing and toileting. And a person with dementia can become incontinent. She may not be able to remember where the toilet is, or react quickly enough to the sensation of needing the toilet.

In the later stages of dementia the person could lose her mobility. She may struggle to walk steadily. She will be more likely to fall over and may eventually be confined to a wheelchair or a bed.

If you decide that you can't care for the person with dementia for whatever reason, don't dwell on it. Work on finding a solution and don't feel guilty. You are doing your best for the person under exceptionally difficult circumstances. The priority is to make sure she receives the care that she needs.

You may want to move the person into a care home. It will of course involve a huge lifestyle change, but in time she should adapt to a new environment. You may question whether she will be happy. It's a difficult question to answer, but if you're sure that things can't go on as they are, then it may be a good solution. A former colleague of mine, who used to visit her granddad in a care home, once said to me: 'You can't necessarily make your mum happy, but you can make her safe.' Those words resonated with me. I knew it was no longer safe for Mum to live alone. And I knew that I couldn't care for her full time. If your parent has reached this stage, the best thing you can do for her is to do your research thoroughly. Make finding the right solution your number one priority.

12

Choosing and paying for a care home

If you are considering moving the person into a care home, don't leave it to the last minute to start the search. The more time you have to do your research, the more likely you are to make the right choice.

At this stage, you may be wondering:

- Who pays for the care?
- What type of care home best suits the person?
- What's the difference between a residential care home and a nursing home?

The laws about who pays for care are different in England, Wales, Scotland and Northern Ireland. There are national rules for each, but also some local variations. However, broadly speaking, wherever you live the process is similar – the local authority (or in Northern Ireland, a health and social care trust) must carry out an assessment of the person's needs. If the person is considered in need of residential care, he may have to contribute towards the cost. In England, Wales and Northern Ireland, the person's financial assets are usually taken into consideration.

So wherever you are in the UK, the first step is to speak to the local authority and ask them to conduct an assessment of the person's needs.

This explanation of how the care system works in England will provide an example of the process – although, as mentioned, there are national variations.

Care in England is not free. Most people will have to pay something towards the cost of their care. The local authority (council) may cover some or all of the cost, but if you are applying for financial help, you need to have the person with dementia assessed by the local authority and they have to agree that the person needs to go into a care home. The person will also be means-tested, which means that what he receives depends on his financial status. If the person has been assessed as needing to go into a care home, and his capital is below £23,250, he should be entitled to financial support. (The value of his home will be taken into consideration.)

The local authority will talk to the person with dementia, and to you as his carer, jointly to produce a care and support plan. This process may have already occurred if the person has been receiving some support at home. After that, the financial assessment will be conducted. The person with dementia or the local authority, or a combination of the two, will pay for care. The means test takes into consideration any income the person receives regularly, such as pensions, stocks, shares and investments, premium bonds and national savings and property. If the person with dementia is living at home alone, he may have to sell his home to pay for care. If his partner is living with him, or an older relative over the age of 60, or a younger adult who is incapacitated, the house will not need to be sold. However, you could also rent out the person's house and use the income to pay for care-home costs.

If the person needs to sell his home, he may get 12 weeks' grace during which time the local authority will foot the bill while the house is being sold. If it's a private care home, the home will usually allow the person to take up a deferred payment scheme, so that he doesn't pay for care until the house is sold.

Can you choose the care home?

If the person is eligible for financial help, then yes, so long as the home is considered suitable for the person's needs and complies with any terms and conditions set out by the local authority. However, it must not cost more than the local authority would normally pay for someone with the same needs. If you have a particular care home in mind that you think is suitable but it is more expensive than the local authority are prepared to contribute, then the authority will allow a third party to top up the fees as long as he or she can afford to keep doing it in the long term. The person is not allowed to top up the fees if his capital is below £23,250. At the time of writing, it has been reported that this threshold will rise from April 2020.

What if the person isn't eligible for funding?

If the person is not considered eligible for local authority funding, he can choose his own care home and pay for the care. He will then be known as a 'Self Funder'. Once the person's capital goes down to £23,250, he can then seek help from the local authority. But if the home costs more than the local authority usually pay, then someone else will need to top up the difference on behalf of the person, or he may need to find alternative care.

Before the person goes into a more expensive care home, take a look at his finances and work out how long his funds will last. It's impossible to predict the future, but if it's likely that the funds will run out before the person dies, then you may need to consider a cheaper care home, or speak to the care home. If the person goes into a more expensive home as a Self Funder, he will be paying more than the local authority would be prepared to pay. You could ask the manager if the home would be willing to accommodate the person at social service funding rates in the long term.

If it reaches the stage where the money runs out and the care home is still charging the same fees, the local authority will take over but may want to move the person to a less expensive care home. However, according to Age UK, the local authority must offer a care home that meets the needs of the person, and you can often argue that there is a compelling need for him to stay in his current home. One argument would be that it would be too disruptive for him to move and potentially risky to his health. You might well be able to argue successfully that the person needs to stay in his current home to meet his needs.

Funded nursing care

The person may already be receiving Attendance Allowance or NHS Continuing Care. If the person is going into a nursing home and is not entitled to NHS Continuing Care, he may be entitled to NHS-funded nursing care if he has a lower level of nursing requirements.

However, this can only be paid to someone living in a care home that is registered to provide nursing care. For more information, visit <www.nhs.uk/chq/Pages/what-is-nhs-funded-nursing-care.aspx>.

Here are some useful links to guides on who pays for care in different parts of the UK:

- England – <www.nhs.uk/Conditions/social-care-and-support-guide/Pages/funding-care.aspx>
- Wales–<http://gov.wales/topics/health/socialcare/care/?lang=en>
- Scotland – <www.scotland.gov.uk/Topics/Health/Support-Social-Care/Financial-Help/Charging-Residential-Care>, and further advice is available from Care Information Scotland on 0800 011 3200 or on the website at <www.careinfoscotland.scot>
- Northern Ireland – <www.nidirect.gov.uk/residential-care-and-nursing-homes>.

In addition, Alzheimer's Society has free downloadable guides to who pays for care in England, Wales and Northern Ireland on its website at <https://www.alzheimers.org.uk> (search under 'Who pays for care?').

Residential home or nursing home?

It's important to distinguish between the two. So what is the difference between a residential care home and a nursing home?

Residential homes

A residential home (also known as assisted living) is for those who can live independently to a certain extent but who need help with some tasks, such as being prompted to eat regular meals or take medication. They may or may not need personal care but may need some supervision to prevent them from getting lost.

The residential care home will provide long-term care and provide residents with hot meals in a communal living area, full housekeeping and laundry services and assistance with personal care, such as washing, dressing and feeding. Those who live in a residential care home can no longer live independently alone, but don't need the amount of care provided in a nursing home. The home will have a schedule of regular activities and social events, such as outings and performers to entertain the residents. A person who can manage some of his own needs may be suited to this environment.

Nursing homes

A nursing home is for those with more complex needs and will have a trained nurse on duty at all times, day and night. It can provide nursing care and manage chronic conditions. Residents will have support with personal care, such as washing, dressing, bathing and feeding if necessary. There will also be regular social activities such as karaoke and wheelchair dancing, and a communal area and a garden.

Which is better?

There is no easy answer to this but, in my view, it's worth seeking advice from the person's GP and mental health team, and also considering not just how he is now but how he may be in the future. Sadly, while it's impossible to guess the rate of future changes, deterioration is likely. Imagine the person with dementia on his worst day, and think about what care he would need on that day.

Finding a good care home

You may have started searching online or perhaps a care home has been recommended to you. I looked at a care home where my friend's father lived as he was very happy there. He liked the home's busy social schedule and enjoyed taking part in activities and going on outings. My mother is not a very social person and prefers quiet time with family and close friends, so this type of home wouldn't have suited her. Her needs were also more complex than those of my friend's father, who was mobile and more independent than my mum. So think about where your parent is now and the help he or she may need, then consider whether the home can meet those needs. Recommendations may not necessarily mean that the home is suitable.

Before visiting a care home you can download the latest inspection report of the home on the Care Quality Commission (CQC) website. The CQC regulates independent care homes (and care agencies) in England and conducts regular inspections to ensure adequate standards are being met. It will look at whether the home is safe, effective, caring, responsive and well led, and will rate the home in each of these categories. You can download and read the report free of charge by visiting the CQC website at <https://www.cqc.org.uk>.

In Wales, the Care and Social Services Inspectorate regulates care homes and the process is similar, though it tends to carry out more unannounced inspections. Visit <www.cssiw.org.uk>.

In Scotland, the Care Inspectorate carries out inspections. Visit <www.careinspectorate.com>.

In Northern Ireland, the Regulation and Quality Improvement Authority regulates care homes. Visit <www.rqia.org.uk>.

Location of the home is hugely important. Ensure it's close to where you live, and easy to reach. This will enable you to visit the person regularly, which will make an enormous difference.

When you have found a few care homes to visit, make an appointment with the manager, so that he or she has time to speak to you and answer questions. When you visit, take note of how the staff treat the residents. Do they speak to them kindly and respectfully? Do they knock on doors before entering residents' rooms? Try to gauge if the home is well staffed.

Does the home smell clean and fresh? I visited a very expensive care home once that had an overpowering stench of urine everywhere. It didn't make a great first impression as I couldn't wait to leave and certainly wouldn't want my mum to live there.

Talk to the residents and ask what they think of the home. You may get a varied response and some may be more able to communicate than others. It's worth speaking to the relatives of people who live at the home too.

Privacy may be important. If your parent is a private person and doesn't like to share bathroom facilities, then ask the care home if he can have his own room with a private bathroom.

Some other points to consider:

- Can his room be personalized? Can he include a few items of his own furniture?

- How much freedom does he have? Can he choose what he wants to wear every day? Can he decide to spend time in his room if the communal area is noisy?
- Can he take any pets with him?
- Does he get a choice of meals? Does each menu have different options? Is he free to eat in his room if he wants to do this?

Dementia training

Ask the home what sort of training the staff have been given. Is it a home that specializes in dementia? What is their policy on coping with challenging behaviour?

My mother is given plenty of time to get up in the morning in her care home. She's never been a morning person, and the staff respect her preference to lie in until late morning. If she refuses to get up, they will leave her in her bed and check on her regularly.

Mobility issues

If the person has limited mobility then ask what provision will be put in place to ensure he isn't at risk of falls. Having a fall will increase the risk of a hospital stay, which can be very distressing for a person with dementia.

Don't overestimate the decor

It's natural that you'll want the person to be in a pleasant environment but it's easy to place too much emphasis on aesthetics. Some care homes pride themselves on offering residents an environment that resembles a hotel. But the most important thing in my view is the level of care the person is receiving, and the interaction he has with the care-home staff.

Practical considerations

Other important considerations include whether the home has wheelchair access as well as a lift, and whether the room is appropriate for the person with dementia. As mentioned, some care homes have shared bathroom facilities, and while this works for some, it may not suit everyone. Some residents would prefer to have their own bathroom.

What's nearby?

It's also important to think about the facilities in and near to the care home. Is there a garden where residents can sit in warmer weather? Is there a nearby shop, restaurant, café or garden centre where you can take the person fairly easily to break up his day?

Is the home secure?

Security is another important factor so that the person with dementia doesn't manage to leave the home and wander off, putting himself at risk. Are the doors locked with special entry codes to gain access?

When can you visit?

Ask the home what their policy is on visits. Are you free to visit any time during the day or evening? Are you free to make a drink for the person and yourself when you visit, and made to feel welcome?

Freedom of choice

When the residents are tired, are they free to go to bed when they want? One care home I visited was understaffed, and I once sat with a dozen tired residents at 10 p.m., who were so exhausted they'd fallen asleep in their chairs. They had given up asking to be taken to bed. The carers were busy putting other residents to bed, but there weren't enough carers on duty to meet everyone's needs.

When you find the right home

If you have found what you think is a suitable home, ask the manager if the person will have a full assessment of his needs. You may also be asked to fill in a document that describes the person, including his family history and likes and dislikes. Ask if each resident has a care plan and how often it gets reviewed.

If you are arranging a home privately, make sure that the home sends you a contract in advance. Read it and ask any questions first. Ask what the notice period is if things don't work out. Make sure you understand how the weekly fees are calculated and how much notice will be given if fees are increased. It's also worth asking what happens if the person's condition deteriorates and whether the home would continue to be able to meet his needs. If not, what alternative arrangements would be made to move him to somewhere more suitable?

More help

For more information on funding, visit:

<www.nhs.uk/Conditions/social-care-and-support-guide/Pages/funding-care.aspx>.

Incidentally, Age UK and Alzheimer's Society both have extensive guides on choosing the right care home on their websites.

13

Life in a care home

When the person first moves into a care home, take a list of all of her medication and the medication itself, along with any other medical records. The care home will have its own GP. You may want to ask the person's existing GP for a printout of her medical records to give to the new doctor. Let the home know if the person has any medical issues, such as a history of heart disease or diabetes, along with any allergies and dietary requirements. The more information you can give the home, the better.

It's also useful to build a picture of the person. Let the care-home staff know about the person's hobbies, her likes and dislikes and what she enjoys. Tell them about anything that will annoy the person or make her happy. Books containing photographs of cats or dogs are guaranteed to make my mum smile on a bad day!

Care homes can sometimes be noisy, so if your parent likes peace and quiet and prefers not to be disturbed too often, it's worth letting the care staff know. She should be entitled to spend more time in her own room if she prefers.

Build a history of the person's life, letting the staff know any details of her spouse and other family members. You may be asked to complete a document with information about the person's life, past and present.

Rob's story
Mum has always liked to watch TV quietly and has never been a fan of noisy environments. She would be the first to complain about the noise in a crowded restaurant. So when she first moved into a care home, she didn't like the afternoons when they would arrange dancing or karaoke, as she found it too noisy. The care-home staff realized that if they settled her into her room with a cup of tea and her favourite TV show for an hour or two, she was much happier, and had the added bonus of someone bringing her cups of tea and biscuits!

Visit regularly

When the person with dementia first goes into a care home, she may be confused about where she is, which may be upsetting but may also be a blessing in disguise. My mother thinks she's in the pub when eating her lunch in the communal room, and this makes her happy.

It may take some time for your parent to settle in and get to know the staff. The more you can visit in the early stages, the better. Let the staff know you are taking her health seriously and care about her greatly.

The person will also do better if you can visit her regularly. If she associates you with feeling safe and secure, then it's natural that she will feel reassured when you visit. You may wonder if there's any point in visiting the person if you think there's a good chance she will have forgotten about your visit a short while later. Think again. A survey by Alzheimer's Society showed that 42 per cent of people stopped visiting relatives who didn't remember the visits. However, the survey also showed that 64 per cent of those with dementia felt isolated from friends and family. Even if the person doesn't remember your visit, she is likely to feel happier afterwards, so don't withdraw. She will feel comforted by familiarity, including the sound of your voice or your smell. Even if she doesn't remember you, your visit will probably have had a positive impact.

Getting involved in social activities offered by the home is a great way to show your support to the staff too. Most care homes have summer barbecues, Christmas parties or occasional dances. If you can attend, it will enhance your parent's enjoyment of the event and let the care home see that you appreciate the job they are doing.

Another good reason to visit the person regularly is that you are letting the care home know that you care about her. You haven't just put her in a home to secure your own freedom; you intend to be a part of her life.

If you are concerned about anything, again, listen to your instincts and make an appointment with the manager. It's the law that all care homes must have a written complaints policy that will tell you whom to contact in the event of a complaint. I would personally recommend trying to build good relationships with care-home staff and management. They will appreciate you visiting the person regularly and the more you get to know them, the more comfortably you can discuss any concerns you may have. In the unfortunate event that you do have to make a complaint that is not dealt with satisfactorily, contact the Local Government Ombudsman (LGO) in England by visiting <www.lgo.org.uk>, in Wales <www.cssiw.org.uk>, in Scotland <www.careinspectorate. com> and in Northern Ireland <www.ni-ombudsman.org.uk>.

You may also want to speak to the Citizens Advice Bureau – visit <www.citizensadvice.org.uk>.

In the right care home, the person can be safe and well, surrounded by others who want to care for her, and hopefully with regular visits from family and loved ones who live close by.

14

A few final thoughts

Living with dementia is extremely tough and if you've taken care of the person and managed to look after yourself in the process, then you've done a great job. It's taught me many valuable life lessons. Caring for my mum has made me more patient and less selfish, and I now value health and happiness above career and money. Even though she doesn't know it, my mum has continued to inspire me and help me understand what really matters.

As you continue to provide care for your loved one, here's a final checklist of some key points to remember:

- You can't do it all on your own – get help and make sure it's reliable help. You need people you can count on.
- The person's moods can change quickly – remember it's not personal if the person with dementia makes nasty comments or becomes aggressive.
- Be prepared to repeat yourself – get used to repeating things, as the person may be unable to remember recent events or conversations.
- Use distraction techniques – if the person is becoming agitated or frustrated, change the subject.
- Don't mention bereavements – if the person asks where deceased relatives are, don't say they've died or your parent will grieve all over again. Distraction techniques may help.
- Routine is important – a change of routine or environment can be very confusing for the person with dementia, so try to stick to his or her usual routine as much as you can and spend time in familiar surroundings.
- Keep an eye on the person's health – if you notice a significant deterioration in your parent's condition, seek medical help and start to plan for how you will continue to meet his or her needs in future.

- Be in a good place – when you visit the person with dementia, make sure you're in a good mood and not too tired or stressed. You have no idea what mood the person will be in when you arrive, so if you can, avoid visiting when you're overtired.
- Look after yourself – take care of your own health for the benefit of both of you.

Useful addresses

Action on Elder Abuse
Tel. (for confidential help): 080 8808 8141
Website: http://elderabuse.org.uk

Age UK
Advice line: 0800 169 2081
Website: www.ageuk.org.uk

The Alzheimer's Show
Website: http://alzheimersshow.co.uk
Annual show offering help and advice for those living with dementia,
with practical advice on its website.

Alzheimer's Society
National Dementia Helpline: 0300 222 1122
Website: https://www.alzheimers.org.uk

Attendance Allowance
Tel. (England, Wales and Scotland): 0345 605 6055
Tel. (Northern Ireland): 028 9090 6178
Website: https://www.gov.uk/attendance-allowance/overview

Care Quality Commission
Tel. (Customer Service Centre): 03000 616161
Website: www.cqc.org.uk
Regulates home-care providers and care homes.

Carehome.co.uk
Website: www.carehome.co.uk/care_search.cfm
A website that will help you find a care home in your area.

Carer's Allowance Unit
Tel. (England, Wales and Scotland): 0345 608 4321
Tel. (Northern Ireland): 028 9090 6186
Website: www.nhs.uk/Conditions/social-care-and-support-guide/Pages/
how-to-claim-carers-allowance.aspx
https://www.gov.uk/carers-allowance

Carer's UK
Advice line: 0808 808 7777
Website: www.carersuk.org
Provides help and advice for carers.

Dementia UK
Helpline: 0800 888 6678
Website: www.dementiauk.org
A national charity with a helpline offering advice for carers and details of
an Admiral Nurse in your area.

NHS England
Website: www.nhs.uk

NHS Northern Ireland
Website: http://online.hcsni.net

NHS Scotland
Website: www.nhs24.com

NHS Wales
Website: www.wales.nhs.uk

Office of the Public Guardian
Tel.: 0300 456 0300
Website: https://www.gov.uk/government/organisations/
office-of-the-public-guardian

Personal Independence Payment
Enquiry line: 0345 850 3322
Website: https://www.gov.uk/pip/overview

United Kingdom Homecare Association
Website: www.ukhca.co.uk/index.aspx

Index